She Rode on Big Charlie (Poems for Mum on Alzheimer's and Dementia)
By Bob Pallister

First edition

All proceeds from the sale of this book will be distributed equally between Alzheimer's Research UK and the Alzheimer's Society.

Introduction

My Mum was the first to know there was something wrong. She had already given up driving after one shunt too many and had been telling me for at least a year she was worried about forgetting things, when her GP sent her for a brain scan in 2014. She was seventy-five. The slightly inconclusive finding was "mild cognitive impairment" and she began attending six-monthly appointments at the Memory Clinic. I would drive her there and sit in on the test where they gave her a score out of 30 for a set series of cognitive and memory tasks. One was to be given a man's name address and remember it two minutes later. He lived in a little town in Devon that we'd visited on holiday in 1969 so the first time she managed to remember the town though not the not the name and got a score of 27/30. Six months later, choose how hard I tried to will the Devon holiday into her brain she didn't get it and got 26/30. This pattern of dropping a point every six months from her score continued for about three years until her diagnosis was upgraded to Alzheimer's.

Meanwhile, working long hours with a mortgage not yet paid I was paying scant attention and assuming Mum was functioning OK. Actually, her world was gradually shrinking. With her inability to remember and keep appointments and her tendency in conversation to repeat what she already said five minutes ago, her social life was dwindling, and lacking the confidence to travel she had stopped going on holiday.

Then I had the great good fortune to be offered voluntary redundancy and the chance to take early retirement with an occupational pension. This enabled me to do two things. One was to pay more attention to my Mum's needs and the other was to reconnect with my youthful love of writing poetry. At first there was very little cross over between these two aspects of my life but gradually Mum and her condition began to appear more and more in what I was writing.

The resulting poems appear in this book in the order in which I wrote them and so closely follow the progress of the condition.

I hesitate to use the word journey because it has become something of a cliché, but I guess that is what this is, our Alzheimer's journey.

Haiku for Mum

House of memories

Doors closed to new visitors

Old ones start leaving

The next poem recalls a hugely important chapter in Mum's life. At the time of writing her long-term memory was still pretty much intact, but my rough understanding was that it would begin to erode, with her childhood, and this scene in particular being the last parts to go

In 24, Limesway

Mum was to my knowledge at the time aged four
When she found her mother asleep on the hallway floor
Nothing she tried to do would bring about her mother's waking
Talking, poking, shouting, even grabbing her and shaking
I remember that hallway from twenty-five years later
When you left the coal fired rooms, the chill couldn't have been
        greater
Somehow around the door frames leaked a draught
That seemed to have the icy fingers of an arctic blast
Thus, Mum's second thought was to keep her sleeping mother
        warm
So, she draped a hearth rug and the doormat over Margot's form
Which satisfied her for a while that she'd done the right thing
But that didn't last long and as more fretfulness kicked in
To knock for help on the next-door semi, she scampered round
Mrs. Powell came straightaway to the hallway and found
The telegram in Margot's hand that had caused the faint and read
"Your husband Flight Sergeant Jack Frankland is missing presumed
        dead"
The reconnaissance flight we later found searched for wreckage
        and survivors
But returned to base disappointed, having found no trace of either
The ripples of that day are still rippling seventy years past

Of all the thing's Mum's going to forget, this will be the last
When all her other memories have into the shadows retreated
There at the end of the corridor on an ironic throne seated
Will be the screen playing that scene of the draughty, cold hallway
In that red brick, semi-detached house at 24, Limesway
Beckoning her back, distracting and impeding her
And in its disembodied way, somehow still needing her

<u>Mum's Memories</u>

One of our repeated conversations
Something that she will tell me all the time
In her head, she's strange, swirling sensations
That she demonstrates with a halo mime
That's the ever-moving waters onto which
Can never settle new memories' fresh snow
No matter how important or how rich
At the moment of touchdown, they will go

<u>Elfchens on Memory I</u>

Reading
My diaries
Helps me remember
How much I have
Forgotten

Forgetting.
The oldest
Memories run deepest
And are hardest to
Dislodge

Family

And friends
Will be our griots
Our storytellers when we're
Gone

Elfchens on Memory II

Our
Lives remembered
As a series
Of anecdotes that we
Embellish

Embellish
Their anecdotes
The others will
About us when we're
Gone

The Memories We Keep I

The dancing thread
Of pictures sped
Inside our heads
A memory-wheel

This projection
Recollection
A connection
We could both feel

Stretched film slackens
Heats and blackens
Flicks off, back on
More flaws revealed

With each new play
There is no way
To make it stay
Perfect and healed

Bit by bit lost
Grown over, mossed
This creeping frost
Her memories steals

Our fleeting dance
No permanence
I take each chance
To spin this wheel

A slow decline
A fog of mind
Each meeting time
More is concealed

A one-way clock
That will not stop
Cannot be dropped
Or else repealed

The Memories we Keep II

I visit each succeeding week
We reminisce, together speak
About our past
Lately I sense they start to seep
From her, those memories we keep
And will not last
In an act of role reversal
For which I've had scant rehearsal
Now she will ask
Me to tell her things about
Her life, that fading in and out
Are hard to grasp

And I try to shine back some light
To distract us both from the sight
Of storm clouds massed

At the time of writing this Haiku, the photo was in a frame in Mum's sewing room and was her most frequently accessed memory. She spent the summer of 1958 working in the bar of Billy Butlin's holiday camp at Filey on the Yorkshire coast, where she spent all her free time hanging around the camp's star attraction, Big Charlie the elephant. Eventually Charlie's mahout Ibrahim (white coat) let her ride him and she spent a whole, happy day perched on his neck.

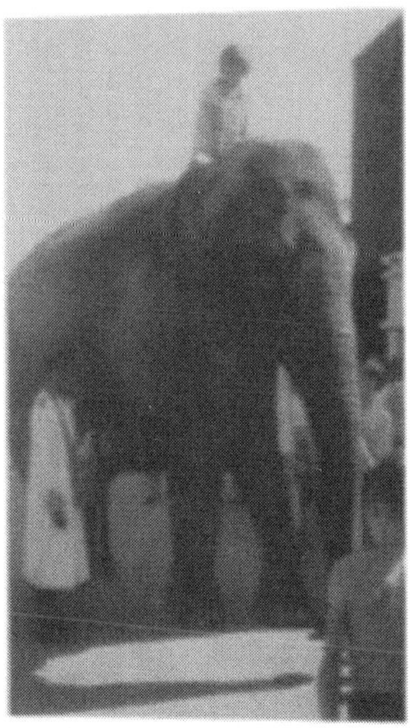

Small life small picture
She's riding on Big Charlie
The largest creature

Shadows

The shadows we cast in our ticking time
Are mercurial and slight
A trick creating our outline
Played by interrupted light
Whereas the shadows that beyond
Our truncated lives we cast
In the hearts of those, of whom we're fond
Will, we hope, their lifetimes last

Elfchen For Mum

Missing
Pieces multiplying
Of her life
As her memories drift
Away

Diminishing Gravity

Now the gravity that fights against the centrifugal forces generated by the spinning of the rock that we were blessed to quite miraculously, randomly and wondrously evolve upon is slowly, sadly, certainly declining for her daily and it's in a losing battle trying to keep her here amongst us and one day we'll all wake up to simply find her flown and gone

For Mum's 80th birthday I whittled this representation of her and Charlie and wrote a sonnet about the two of them

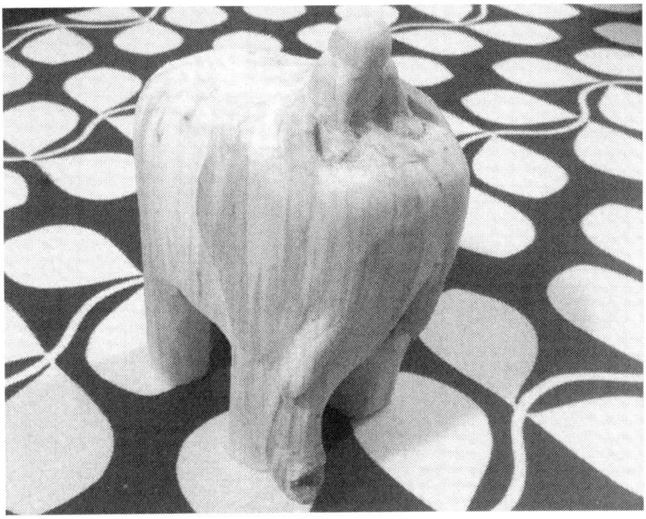

Sonnet for Big Charlie

A zoetrope of memories revolving
A gradually thinning out array
Looming larger while the others are dissolving
Big Charlie who once carried her all day

Whose ears caressed her legs to hold her steady
That summer she worked Billy Butlin's bar
Nineteen, and for her whole life almost ready
Are our memories who we were or who we are?

With Ibrihim and Charlie on Filey's sand
A squirted trunk full of the cold North Sea
Like a water cannon so she could not stand
Up, which like children, brought to them both glee

These are the scenes her zoetrope's rewinding
While other stuff gets lost, she'll always find him

The Ripples We Leave

Grandad Jack is still "missing, presumed dead"
Somewhere in the Gulf of Lyon, the blue waters of the Med'
That's the way the telegram was worded to arrive, as
The reconnaissance mission found no trace of wreckage or survivors
Too much disturbance in the water in 1944 to tell
Where the ripples' widening circles were, that could show them where he fell
In 2019, though I can't locate their epicentre
The ripples are visible yet in a world I can still enter
When I look into my mother's life and eyes and see
A longing for a different narrative that could never come to be
A stark silhouette of absence stands there still
That by an old shoe-box full of letters can't be filled
Addressed to his children, to be, by their mother read aloud
Scant lost pieces of this lost jigsaw that are all she was endowed
With a couple of photographs and a fine little pencil sketch
An abruptly shortened story deprived of a gentler "what's next!"
My mother's memories are fading but these ripples still have the force
To draw her so far back from now to the impact of their source

Mum's Life in The Moment

Mum's calendar's obsolescence
It took me a while before the penny dropped
It's like a railway timetable in essence
In a world where every clock has stopped

No help at all, with now's reference point not known
Just a random series of departures
The leaving ripples of a large rock thrown
Dissipating through the station's arches

Over the shoulder of her permanent today
Is nothing but an ever-thickening mist
That swallows whole each succeeding yesterday
And across tomorrow starts to drift

Unanchored from chronology, her days
Resemble ever more closely her cats'
Patrol the garden in repeating ways
Sleep and eat and wash and more sleep catch

Life in the moment is her shrinking world
So little story left to be unfurled

My earliest memory of my Mum

A Memory in Haiku

Sudden barking dog
Fearful toddler's heartbeat booms
Calmed in mother's arms

In 1944 (Told in Poetic Sandwich)

On the afternoon sofa she wakes
She feeds the cats but not herself
She recognises one by one
The photos on her shelf
Today the day, the date, the time all quite unknown

Her mother was laid asleep on the hallway floor
She had difficulty waking her
She was at the time the age of only four
She tried pinching, she tried shaking her
Where her shallow breathing Mum had been
discovered
It was cold in the hallway so she fetched
The front room hearth rug, and tenderly, Mum
covered
An image in her mind forever etched
Time passed; her mum was warm but not roused yet
Laying oblivious still on the hallway floor

She left for help in a growing sense of fret
Her frightened fist reached up to knock at next door's
door
The neighbour came to see; the paper in mum's hand
She read "... missing presumed dead"; official
telegram

Cats fed she does some dusting
Some adjusting of each curtain
Though her memories are mercurial now
This one keeps coming back for certain
That day, that date, will time begin to smudge?

In his early 80s my paternal grandfather suffered a stroke that left him with aphasia (a loss of language and vocabulary). Unable to get to the end of a sentence without stopping at a word he could no longer find this made the last years of his life frustrating and isolated. The French poet Charles Baudelaire (1821-1867), of whom I'm a bit of a fan, suffered an even worse stroke aged only 45 which left him with no power of speech at all for his last year alive.

Lost for Words (Baudelaire's Final Year)

The voluptuous markings of quill on the page
The voluptuous soundings of words on the tongue
To aphasia lost, forty-five years of age
That part of brain function gone, stroke-struck and
stung
In brothels and gambling dens, syphilis shared
Opium, alcohol; both taken to gird
A soul that in downcastness often despaired
Charles Baudelaire was in love with the word
That could lift the mundane, making magical scenes
Could weft and weave tapestries out of the grime
A fantastic filigree, nightmares, and dreams

An expression of everything, life, death, and time
Time he could quicken by thinking in language
One blood vessel burst and all of that stopped
No therapy, no cure, not even a bandage
Into a corrupt file every single bit locked
Every word, every phrase, every tongue that he'd
learned
In a Babel of silence, both out and both in
Locked from a world where he never returned
And unravelling his thoughts couldn't even begin
His mind in held doldrums of absolute still
The albatross shot, no rewriting the plot
Crawled through his last year with nothing to fill
The hole where his poetry now simply was not

In Her Evanescent Years

A hymn in distant school hall pricks the ears
A photograph in pigtails that was her
A long-lost following of counted years
What day it is today become a blur
The past, a guest, less frequently appears
Between the things that are and things that were

A lost delineation, as it were
Some melodies will never leave the ears
But pictures of the singers start to blur
An empty decade built on fullest years
A shrinking world, a pair of cats and her
Old photographs in which she still appears

Uncertainty about how it appears
Begun to spread to how she thought they were
Increasingly confusing to her ears
The news each day a weak and scrambled blur
A slower life, a speeding up of years
A thinning, dwindling life surrounding her

Those felines, two, that sleep as much as her
Still sleeping every day when sun appears
Each sleep erasing more of how things were
Two languid cats, two pairs of twitching ears
The day, the month, the year, always a blur
Her story at a stand now many years

Her age no longer known, how many years
Familiar becoming weird to her
An odd song that can spook forgetful ears
A cracked mosaic of glimpses, how things were
What she sees every day now strange appears
A story out of focus now a blur

Rain on a watercolour makes it blur
A mystery, an unknown count of years
The timeline of her life evading her
A bus stop where no service now appears
A place where no things are but many were
Sibilance barely audible to ears

What's left of her, her outline disappears
Lost in a blur, her evanescent years
To how they were, won't go back it appears

"So Please Remember This"

In lesson time we watch the watch
With its hands creeping notch by notch
As time goes by
There's no wind in our spirit's flag
As we sit bored and watch it drag
As time goes by
Next working on the hamster wheel
We sell it by the hour's the deal
As time goes by
We film the action, others play

We're making memories they say
As time goes by
Who were those faces? We forget
Where were those places? We forget
As time goes by
With all the futures that we planned
All passed like water through our hands
As time goes by
From summit, panoramic view
Of all the climbing we went through
As time went by
Pray memories, clouds don't roll across
And all our hard-earned view's not lost
Of time gone by

Relocation Triggered

Melting the electric kettle on the gas ring was a bad sign
But you rage at the pill dispenser, that little gadget trade named Tab Time
Proved the bigger problem and though I resealed it when I'd put all the batteries back
At the sound of its alarm, it was trashed and binned again in your very next attack
And so, a daily visit to dole out your medication
Was the trigger for your move, your nearer me relocation

Photos showing the erosion of Anne Bronte's grave stone in Scarborough Church yard over recent years

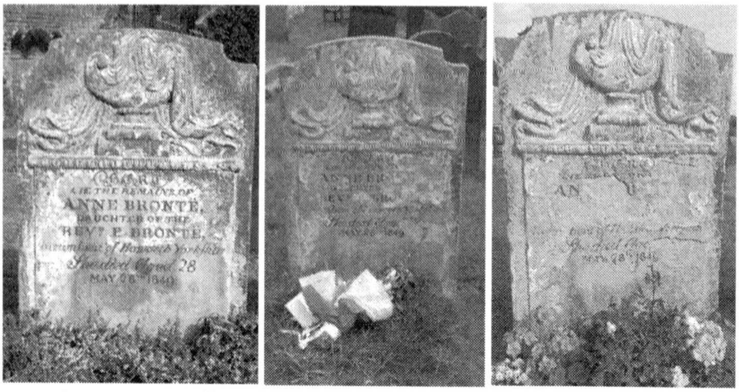

Mum's Memories (Like Anne Bronte's Headstone)

Each day there's more escaping
Mum's present form forsaking
Her memories called home
Lost track of earth's revolving
All dates and time dissolving
Like acid rain-washed stone

By Scarborough Church Anne Bronte's
Stone mason chiselled font is
Now smoothed to stony skin
A new blue sign that's placed there
Now indicates the space where
Anne Bronte lies within

Sort pills and bills and feed her
And every day I read her
Life story from a book
Re-chiselling her bare stone
To help her feel she's there home
With who she is lit up

Death, my Grandma invited
So she'd be reunited

With my Dad, her belief
Maybe they're waiting up there
Mum's memories out somewhere
With Time's repentant thief

Her soul, her whole life story
A crazy idea for me
To join them up once more
Meanwhile I just remind her
Of all the life behind her
And who she was before

A Short Song for Mum

She's lost her life-story, it's just leaked away
So I've written it down for her, and we read it each day
There are three places where it makes her laugh
Each time as fresh-funny as it was the last
Each laugh-recognition, each transient spark
Is a small consolation, small light in the dark
And though Mum thinks her Mum's still living,
    she's always pleased to find
It was she who read her eulogy.
This gives her peace of mind

Question Time

Suspended always in the now
No future plans no past to know
Though you still know the code by which
The hands that crawl around your watch
Should help you find your place in time
The watch you wear because you wear it, not for any helpful
    reason
A habit like the handbag carried with no money now or keys in

Always the trigger for two queries
"Is this watch wrong or is it right?"
And the second in the series
"Then is it day or is it night?"

Nao Was Still the Matriarch

Nao was still the matriarch when we took her to the vet
With loud and laboured breathing and in obvious distress
A tumour on her lungs was the diagnostic call
And euthanasia a kindness was agreed by you and all
Nao was your twelfth cat and your instincts still ran deeper
Than in pain and suffering to think to try to keep her
And I never shared your love of pets, I missed out on that gene
But found it was my job that day to stand and watch the scene
With you as Nao lay there with still dark and lustrous fur
On that table as the needle very gently did for her
And her glassy eyes stayed open as to nought her breathing tailed
I stared into their emptying, by sadness great assailed
I'd always found your cats annoying and your love for them a quirk
But the stoic one that day was you, I don't know how that works
Back in the back garden it was burial at dusk
I did all the digging and did all I though we must
Benny soon got used to not waiting to eat second
But mostly got called Nao each time he was by you beckoned

Benny's Bowl

What's in benny's bowl today? I'm frequently nonplussed
He'll eat the mini-pork-pies' meat, though always leaves the crust
While yoghurt, quiche and Weetabix all meet with his disgust
Rice pudding, grapes, tomatoes, half a macaroni cheese
Or bits of chopped banana, I find he's keen on none of these

I wrote it in block capitals, the 'CAT FOOD' label on the drawer
But you always look surprised each time I point out what it's for

It's Still Me!

There's a little book we wrote
        about the story of your life
You laugh three times each time we read it
        never only once or twice
And it's always the same laughter
        and it's always the same places
It brings, I see it clear in yours
        a little light to both our faces
It's a message from the wilderness
        from all you used to be
Saying not to worry
        "I'm still here and it's still me!"

No Movement Class

She was lying on the rug like a tiny tin soldier when I arrived today
The dusk was falling and the lights were out and when I asked, I heard her say
"I'm doing a movement class but I must be doing it wrong because everyone's gone away"
And it was true enough, there was only me
But maybe I could've joined her class
Maybe I could've *been* her class
But soon enough the moment passed
And light switched on I microwaved her tea

Stolen Memories

She sleeps longer than a teenager and quieter than a cat
Curtains closed from early evening till midday
In each long, peaceful silence in a riot of an act
A few more of her memories are stolen clean away
Her walls are filled with family photographs, I tell her
all their names
Sometimes she smiles at the reminder, sometimes
it's like she didn't know
I'm stranded like Canute against this relentless tide
of change
Watching each sandcastle memory get stolen by
the dark, in-creeping flow

Vision Vanquished

At first you took to jigsaws, great! No memory required,
all the pieces on the table, out before you, out to see
and in the now
But as I did them with you, I began to find that more
and more the bits that fit were found by me to your
surprise
Like all the helpful sticky labels I'd stuck on the drawers
and cupboards that you'd not noticed when I pointed
to somehow
And you could only find the cat food when you were
looking for the tea bags, I'd show the pictures of the
cats upon the boxes and you'd nod, but I'd not know
how this world looked now to your eyes
First it was time that was defeated as the past became a
blur and the future disappeared into haze you couldn't
plan for, just the present left, a doldrums where you
languished

Then the view began to leak out its connections of
cognisance, not enough that memory's routed, now
seems vision must be vanquished

(after Alan Bennett's Auntie)
These concern a story I read about the writer Alan Bennet's Auntie. She had Alzheimer's and absconded from her care home wearing only her nightie and slippers one evening. Her family were alerted and Alan's brother ended up in the unenviable position of being the one who found her, lying dead from hypothermia in the nearby woods the following day. This story haunted me when my Mum began her episodes of "wandering".

Their Lost Auntie

A journey into wayward woods
A lost sense of direction
A frost had blasted all the buds
A journey into wayward woods
They searched and searched it was no good
She defied all their protection
A journey into wayward woods
A lost sense of direction

The Last of All Her Trials

They went looking for her in the woods in Weston-super-Mare
She had slippers on, a dressing gown, grey tousled curly hair
She was answering a restless call to find something she'd forgotten
The lanes, the fields, the hedgerows, they searched from top to
bottom
It was hypothermia that took her, overnight amongst the trees
Her slippered feet through leaf mold misdirected by degrees
Of her growing inner struggle to connect with knowledge files
Which that night proved insurmountable in the last of all her trials

Listicle of Lifetimes for Mum

In one lifetime you rode an elephant, Big Charlie and you bathed him on the beach and got cannoned for your trouble by a trunk full of North Sea

In another lifetime you found you mother lying unconscious in the hallway; you were four and draped a rug on her to help her in some small way, didn't know her faint was caused by the telegram that read that her Flight Sargent husband had been posted 'missing, presumed dead'.

Who in yet another lifetime had brought home for you, a kitten in the pocket of his overcoat, it's true, she got Judy as her name, and through all your other lifetimes, your love of cats would remain.

In another lifetime again you found tied to the bars of his hospital cot, your one-year-old son's wrists and that made you very angry, and though you never forgave or forgot, you very quickly got his hands free.

In another lifetime you packed picnics in the boot of the car, pâté and camembert to eat by the River Loire.

In another lifetime you sewed all your small boys' clothes, new ones needed every year, how quickly small boys grow!

In another lifetime, from marriage and parenthood freed, you learned all the words with the operatic society, "wouldn't it be love-er-ly!" indeed.

In another lifetime they promoted you to head teacher above, but you never really liked it, being with little ones in the classroom had been the job you really loved.

In another lifetime still, you rang bells in your church, where somehow your tiny arthritic wrists withstood the bell rope's lurch.

Now all of those lifetimes are still yours but are hidden or hard to find, and the best I can do every day is to share my scrapbook mind.

Her Dad's Final Letter

Her Dad's final letter
We read it yesterday
Wrote he hoped to be home
To see her fifth birthday
He never made it there
Last resting place at sea

Missing presumed dead
"So, who's my Dad now?"
She asked me, confused
Seventy-seven
Whole years have gone by

Today I found
In kitchen bin
Torn to pieces
Her Dad's letters

Rescued them.
Another
Unwanted

Milestone
Left her

Home

For Her, The Familiar and Unfamiliar Blur

Walking her to our house for sharing Sunday tea
"Have I been to your house?" she always asks of me
"Hundreds of times!" I say, she looks but doesn't see
"I lived here once, didn't I!" sure as she could be
I always say she didn't; perhaps I should agree

The familiar and unfamiliar blur
There are no certainties left graspable for her

She'd set off for the corner shop, carrying there
A tiny suitcase like Paddington Bear
A passing Good Samaritan became aware
Found an address on her suitcase, drove her right there
To find new folks had moved in, her quite unaware

The familiar and unfamiliar blur
There are no certainties left graspable for her

I picked her up from the headquarters of police
There, sitting drinking tea, her feet up on a seat
Charming all the officers, her compliments sweet
The men are all "So tall!" she'll many times repeat
The women all have "lovely hair" and "kept so neat"

The familiar and unfamiliar blur
There are no certainties left graspable for her

Her second walkabout, we're away not there
A one-thirty AM knock gives our son a scare
Out from a police car with her shock of grey hair
His confused grandmother is transferred to his care
When asked where she'd been and why, she isn't aware

The familiar and unfamiliar blur
There are no certainties left graspable for her

A third wander in the rain on Halloween night
More Good Samaritans found her, she was alright
The back door key I'd chained to her door frame, screwed tight
She wore round her neck, my best laid plans thwarted. Quite!
So now I've bought her her "James Bond tracking device"

The familiar and unfamiliar blur
There are no certainties left graspable for her

Mum's New house

Every morning
Same question
Whose house is this?

Repeating
Confusing
Unfamiliarity
Feeling of unbelonging

Silent Forgiveness

We were neither of us perfect as mother or son
All the dysfunctional stuff in my youth that was done
At all the wrong times, the wrong things that we said
I thought I couldn't forgive you till we were one of us dead
But with you now, all I see is a person in need
And in two so different ways, from our pasts we're both freed

Till Winter Fades

I'll wait for you till
Winter fades
And stealthy brutal
Slow decades
Strip bare the branches
One by one
Of all the dances
That we've done
To leaf mould on
The forest floor
Like we're no longer
Here no more
Our evanescent
Presence fades
Forgotten lessons
Choices made
A smudge of ochre
Underfoot
When Autumn's over
Winter's up
And Spring belongs to
Other birds
Our echoes maybe
Stay behind
To bring us vaguely
Back to mind

The Universe Outside Mum's Windows

Her watch
In suspicion
She reads and doubts it
Always "is that really the time?
Is it morning or night?"
No appointments
To keep
Her calendar
Long out of use now joined
By the watch she still wears and checks
Out of ingrained habit
To say but not
To know
But just to be
To sleep to wake to doze
To eat to sleep to watch to wait
Closer kindred to the cat she's always kept
Except that feline Benny can find his way home
His homing instinct unsmudged by his years
Here where a gentle letting go
And gentle clinging on
Both intertwine
Night falls
And sun rises
Random inhalations
And the rhyming exhalations
The Universe outside
Is still making
While here
Inside her home
The story's in the book
The pages are getting dog eared
And I'm the last one left
That can read it
To her

Her Reality's Retreated

Her reality's retreated to a half-known dreamlike state
She can't trace how she's been placed here, glimpse no series of
events
Like a dream without a waking up, no sunrise to make sense
While time's concept's something she can't even guess or estimate
When? Where? Questions she can't answer make her night-time
anxious, tense
Her reality's retreated to a half-known dreamlike state
This unanchoredness, uncertainty, she can't elucidate
I detect it in her eyes sometimes, it always gives a wrench
She can't follow her own story now, blurred future, no suspense
Her reality's retreated to a half-known dreamlike state

In The Space Between Now and Forever

The space between now and forever is small
A gap we can barely perceive
But that's where she's lived since this malady called
In fuggy today with her narrative stalled
Past lost where it can't be retrieved

The storybook closed to her that was her life
No page the next chapter to write
I typed her biography, printed and spliced
With photos from scrapbooks on precious advice
It brings back a flickering light

She laughs in three places, the same three each time
As we read together her book
All previous readings all gone from her mind
It's fresh and brand new to her each time I find
By small consolation I'm struck

Her walls full of pictures, I tell her their names
Her grandchildren caught as they grew
Who she thinks is who, no two days is the same
It varies, the access to files in her brain
Despite all my triggers and clues

Some days her granddaughters, she thinks they are her
Her age always seems a surprise
The who that she is and the family we were
Her focus each day more and more of a blur
I see when I look in her eyes

Collapsing time and defeating death

When the social worker calls and she's assessed
Mum's worries for another are repeatedly expressed
"But what are we going to do about Granny Turnbull? Where's
she's going to live?"
She comes back to this question every time
Although when Granny Turnbull died it was still nineteen-forty-nine

What's In a Name?

My benign, familiar face, she sees it, every day
Who am I? to her though, perhaps her brother,
long estranged
Twenty-five years, since their Mum's funeral, yet I get David,
that's his name

Devious Dream-Mind

By her devious dream-mind dread death's been defeated
All of time's been collapsed and the Reaper's been cheated
Whatever heat-scorched and stuttering, flickering film
She can still rescue from her memory's kiln
Choose however distant all who might appear
If she can still see these dream-scenes they must still be here
Her Dad's youthful death I thought could never leave her
But now without my reminders it's getting lost in this fever

It's Chopped Down Her Family Tree

A jumbled jigsaw in a biscuit box upon a high shelf kept
That's where I'll find her family tree all broken down and swept
She's no longer sure which piece I am or where her and I fit
And can't remake it by herself unless I help her bit by bit
Most occasions when she hears who's who, sweet recognition rises
But as time's passed it's grown ever more for her, a story of surprises

Life's Not Quite Perfect Full Circle

When our children were tiny, their milestones came fast
And at each one they needed us less than the last
When the roles are reversed, each slight change from before
Tells the child that the parent now needs them some more

The Ripples Have Almost Stilled Now

I thought the ripples from her father's death could only finally stop the day his daughter died
Could not imagine they might pre-decease her and upon her loving watch simply subside
But now I stand before the sea the bitter blackened sun of this disease has gone and dried
I find it baked to mud its motion ceased, all memory's threads now left in shreds, her past denied

One cold February night the brilliant Telecare team who monitored Mum's bungalow door rang me at 0100 to tell me her door alarm had gone off but they couldn't get her to answer. I checked my App for the "James Bond tracking device" acquired through the Alzheimer's Society that I keep hidden in her handbag. It told me the device was still in the bungalow. Assuming she'd just been letting the cat in I went up to check the door was locked. The back door was indeed unlocked and Benny the cat was snoozing on top of the empty bed over the headboard of which hung Mum's handbag. I rang 999 and quoted the 'Herbert Protocol'. The police were brilliant and found her within the hour, nearly two miles away, walking in her slippers with a dressing gown over her nightie. Haunted by the story of Alan Bennett's Auntie, I kept mum locked in for the week it took me to get her the place in respite care in the care home was to become her next home. It was precisely twelve months after I'd moved her into the bungalow to be closer to me for my daily visits.

No Sugar-Coated Ending

I woke up this morning with one half of me relieved
That I no longer have to care for you but the other half felt
bereaved
You walked your burden off my shoulders, you walked out of my
grasp
But you couldn't tell me to where or why, was futile of me to ask
It's leaving me behind, this journey of your brain
It's now taken you past halfway to some other-world domain
A frustrated sense of failure mixed with relief and grief and guilt
Now you've dismantled every last one of the precautions that I'd
built
I want a sugar-coated ending; I want Phoenix wings to span
But the best that I can manage is 'I've done the best I can'

Captain Oates in Slippers

A waking after midnight in a dream state
Unable to pinpoint your when or where
This bed, this house, this life which ones were yours?
The darkness doesn't help it doesn't seem late

To your questions could the answers be out there?
The thought then, clicked into motion, did you pause?
Captain Oates, but in your dressing gown and slippers
When you left Benny's Captain Scott warm on your bed
I wonder if you left him your best wishes
And "I won't be long" or "I may be some time" what you said

Thoughts on Going into a Care Home

Her new companions merely shadows and pale ghosts of who they were
This is the destination to whose care you do refer

Paraphernalia you'd not used for years and would not use again
And I'd failed to find a home for came to its angry end
As I threw it in the council skip so hard I hurt my arm
But nobody turned to ask me and nobody took alarm
And I put the rear seats back up and I drove home empty booted
Not everything we let go can somehow be substituted

Downsized to a bungalow, then left it for a care home, it's bereavement by degrees
All this emptying of houses, all these melancholy moments that result from your disease

The Music of an Emptying House

My sorrow like music in strange patterns played
As I emptied her house
Of the things she embroidered, the doll's clothes she made
As sorrow like music in strange patterns played
For her talents and skills by decay all betrayed
By sleeping draft doused

And all I could do was keep busy and hum
"...my sunshine, you are..."
With all of the clues as to who was my Mum
Was all I could do to keep busy and hum

And not stop to think, just to get the job done
No door left ajar

Ask what had she done in a year living here?
Her life stuck on hold
No new stories made, old ones just disappeared
Say what had she done in her year living here?
How is she today? I don't know but it's clear
This chapter will fold

Back into a page of invisible ink
All straightaway lost
Not one scene shot here she'll reflect on or think
About just a page of invisible ink
For me though I try, I just cannot resync
Her year here embossed

Of my daily visits whose list of tasks grew
As her powers shrank
And each one she lost she could never renew
While my daily visits, its list of tasks grew
Imperceptible nightfall, life's dark evening drew
To erase the page blank

At one in the morning my nine-nine-nine call
Made next to her bed
Left empty to wander: my safe-built nest's fall
At one in the morning, that nine-nine-nine call
In slippers and nightie, found by police trawl
Asked why, just shook her head

"Crossing the bar" is a nautical expression referring to the 'sandbar' that collects at the point where a river opens out into the ocean. Alfred, Lord Tennyson (1809-1892) used it for the title of a famous short poem.

For Mum, After Tennyson's 'Crossing the Bar'

I

You only got a mile and a half
It wasn't all that far
But it took my best-hatched plans apart
That night you crossed the bar

II

I thought you were safely anchored in the harbour
Until that silent tide rose higher lifting you
Up and out across the bar then farther, farther
The sight of us behind lost from your drifting view
And I know there is no rescue craft to launch
And neither wind or tide will float you home
But so seaworthy is the vessel that has borne
You I could not guess for how long out there you will roam

After a year of thinking I was doing the right thing keeping Mum living "independently" in her own home, I was struck by how much less anxious and how much calmer and more contented she seemed surrounded by other people in her care home.

To Keep Her Soul Afloat

The things we left behind
Now seldom come to mind
Important as they seemed the day we left
My diary: hopes and fears
I saved it all these years
Now never opens up and I feel blessed
Are they less precious than we thought?
All of those memories, did we carry them for nought?

Her independence gone
Some of her light once shone

Has come back since the final petals dropped
Released all from the trees
Each seed blown by the breeze
Will make a life choose where it settles stopped
Now her contented calm I note
Perhaps just to be's enough to keep her soul afloat

The Things We Left Behind

The things we left behind
Less often come to mind
As Earth rotates
The tides won't stay
And ebb away
Just as the moon dictates

Each day the beach washed clean
No evidence we've been
No written names
No words persist
Of lovers' trysts
Our glories or our shames

These castles made of sand
These lives built by our hand
Are sharp as glass
More fiercely sensed
And more intense
For knowing they will pass

'Dylan's night' at the end of the next poem refers to the famous Dylan Thomas poem "Do Not Go Gentle into That Good Night".

Our Finite Night

Hope my past will last
Pictures in my head
Not be fading fast
Who was in the cast
Dimmed each night in bed

Keep them there to share
Knowing who is I
It's a simple prayer
Passing time please spare
Memories in my eye

Take not heart apart
Leave me with the sense
Of a followed chart
Of an end and start
As some recompense

For my finite night
Spent upon this ride
Moon my way to light
At the time seemed bright
Now it turns the tide

Morning's break awake
Will it all be gone?
Numbness or an ache?
Thirst that I can slake
Silence or a song?

Fret nor frown for crown
Struggle not nor fight
Merciful the sound
Gentle she'll go down
Into Dylan's night

A Walk with Mum

A walk round the park in the springtime
Where you take my arm, I'm your guide
See children up onto their swing climb
Or skateboards or scooters to ride
No sign to those passing how dwindled
The light in your mind that once shone
You've, choose how I try to keep kindled
No sense of what's gone

The toddlers by hands being led round
Know more of who they are than you
The truth that I'm getting my head round
About which there's nought I can do
Contentment comes easy, small pleasures
When babies and dogs you look on
Yet over fast past, fleeting treasures
No sense of what's gone

A tea in the café and teacake
You've walked a long way, not complained
Not a word of fatigue or of feet ache
Our small talk's all sweet and restrained
Kids, dogs that we see repetition
We over and over speak on
But me being not a magician
No sense of what's gone

Caring Passed

Who will my visits serve
If you forget me?
Would I my duties swerve
If you just let me?
A question I avoid
Up till when I am buoyed
That you seem overjoyed
By greeting words

For me you were my task
You gave me purpose
My swan legs moving fast
Beneath the surface
Now storm and pond are stilled
No nesting site to build
My duties done fulfilled
These things don't last

Mum Staying Mum

Out of everybody, that I have ever known
She was always amongst, the most accident prone
With a scar on one leg, from a dropped paving stone
And one on one forearm, where they pin-fixed the bone

That break came from a slip, on a fresh-polished floor
Then there was her grabbing, that runaway car door
At first running then dragged, to catch-stop it before
A tree did the stopping, with her dragged legs blood-raw

She once used some scissors, a live-wire to sever
Got thrown with a flash, when the blades came together
Bounced up as surprised, as if floored by a feather
Melted scissor handles, she just shrugged whatever

All her fearlessness, recklessness, bubbled within
That day not to be phased, by a full wheelie-bin
She climbed on it to pogo, to get more crammed in
Result; one broken arm, and a gash on her chin

So the day that her care-home, staff telephoned me
And explained that they had to, it's "policy" see
But Mum dragged a table, to the wall and then she
Climbed and stood on it, to get the window catch free

To get it closed because, she was feeling a draught
That was so recognisably her, I just laughed
That so gung-ho approach, to the needs of the task
Risk-blind and impulsive, her old nature still cast

Nearly 83

Photographs of Mum's granddaughters
She sometimes mistakes as ones of her
When I tell her her life story
The simplest numbers are now a blur
Two children, three grandchildren
Though both news to her she'll take my word
But her age of nearly 83
She really doubts, it's so absurd!

An Acrostic Italian Sonnet on My Mum

My eyes meet hers, the light of recognition's
Unmistakable, I see it every time
Mind you, if pressed who I am, she can't find

How we are related, my position
A stab is made, constrained by her condition
So as her brother David I'm defined

Despite estrangement, decades long resigned
Expired, alive? Lost track of his condition
My ritual of trawling through her pictures
Elicits names and places she's forgot
Never twice the same what she remembers
The flicker of her recall has no fixtures
In adult life, few characters, no plot
And every time a little more surrenders

It Took so Long for it to Cease to Matter

There's a story in between us that you never understood
I've never put my point of view but one day I thought I would
And I'd never quite forgiven you, and I never thought I could
I thought when you got near the end, I might tell you how I felt
I thought then I'd explain where I was sure the blame all dwelt
But then the Gods of irony, their shuffle-skewed hand dealt

Shredding all your memories of the narrative between us
Your adult life a fading blur, both love and misdemeanours
Unsure just who I am to you, you can't revisit or relive this
Which has drained all of my appetite for withholding my forgiveness

<u>In Answer to Dylan Thomas's 'Do Not Go Gentle into That Good Night'</u>

They talk of 'battling' or of 'fighting', well that's not what I wish for you
Your old "no resuscitation" letter tells me you don't wish it too
After life's challenges and gifts, after all that you've been through
Let your embers flicker down to a tiny crimson dot
Balmed by an idle breeze and released from being hot
Just a pinprick on a finger that can smudge a last full stop
In a moment of neutrality, regrets and rage forgot
When a life ends in old age with a long-completed plot
Page after later page, blank, just a number at the top
It's a time for sharing memories, crying tears I will try not
As the poet never said, into that good night gently slide
Your adventures all built-castles washed to smooth beach by the tide
And if I can but be there for you, both together we'll abide

<u>Still Going Gentle</u>

Your sliding into that good night is so cat languid slow and gentle
That my rage against the dying of your light now seems almost incidental
Dances danced, deeds done, songs sung, retreat into the echo
A clenched fist once young now like a flower just opens up to let go

<u>"Do Not Resuscitate" Order</u>

Please keep her comfortable, please do everything to can to
But it's impossible that she might miss a future she can't plan for

Team Spirits

Pressed in the pages of your albums are the pictures of the people that we were that we became before we weren't
This jumbled jigsaw of the pieces of the choices and the chances and the changes contributing to the things that we've forgotten we once learnt
All the hockey teams and netball teams and swimming teams of youth
It's now random who you point to when I ask which one was you

Taking My Word

You may not recognise your photograph and think that others are you
But you'll tend to take my word for it, lost the confidence to argue

Birthday Out

And every time I turn around to see why you have stopped
You're either picking up the litter that somebody else has dropped
Or complimenting someone's baby or admiring someone's dog
No control over what random things will next grab your attention
To not lose you requires vigilance, there's no magical prevention
One son and two grandchildren, there were three of us in charge
But all three got distracted and you ended up at large
After your birthday walk, we took you on through the park to the café
We were dawdling in the churchyard, that was where you got away
Down a centuries old stone staircase by the wall and up the hill
"Who was watching Grandma?", three blank looks, one collective chill
Split up in three directions each one scurrying to find you
Fifteen minutes I spot you far ahead and I'm hurrying behind you
You were slogging dogged up the slope, no notion to where bound
And oblivious what the fuss was for when you were caught and found

The Baby Dolls

Random babies from the communal crib on your dresser keep collecting
"Other people keep grabbing them and they're mine!" is not the answer I'm expecting
When I gently suggest we put them back
But ownership's a tricky concept when you can't remember where you got things
And your squabbles over these babies have been reported by staff watching
Describing the man whose arm you punched and the lady who you slapped

Remembrance Sunday

Remembrance at the cenotaph, we sang the National Anthem
The ritual was good for you, it brought a little back
Familiar words and symbols; brief small mercies seem to grant them
Like recalling who your father was if not who you became from that

A Photograph of Us

Choose what tomorrow was when we were young
The distant present's left it far behind
A boy stands pointing at the setting sun

Behind him, silhouetted watching, Mum
He's almost unaware he's in her mind
Choose what tomorrow was when we were young

The drifting echoed notes of songs we sung
Pass on the breeze, still heard but half-defined
A boy stands pointing at the setting sun

Connections near unravelled, near undone
Our drifting stars felt often misaligned
Choose what tomorrow was when we were young

The circle's grown so wide now, almost run
The boy's become the one that stands behind
A boy stands pointing at the setting sun

By unsought circumstance this picture hung
Upon the wall beside the now drawn blind
Choose what tomorrow was when we were young
A boy stands pointing at the setting sun

When challenged to write a "nice" Halloween poem about a 'Benevolent spirit', the said spirit turned out to owe a little bit to Alan Bennett's auntie and a lot to my Mum

Her Benevolent Spirit

My phone lost its signal, the battery went dead
With thick clouds and sunset, deep darkness soon spread
The wind it was restless, tree branches it whipped
While drizzle, relentless off all their leaves dripped
The path lost in darkness, no landmarks to see
I swore I heard footsteps come following me
Adrenaline-fueled heartbeat raced, I was swift gripped
By fear and I ran but soon stumbled and tripped
I sensed a faint glow and looked up to behold
A softly lit face that was wrinkled and old
Framed by grey hair like the twigs of a nest
In slippers and night dress I sensed she was dressed
She gazed down, spoke gently "there's nothing to fear
Like you I got lost the first time I came here
I was searching for all of the memories I'd lost
I found them but finding them came at a cost

And they buried the part of the me that they found
But the memories stayed here, they are not in the ground"
She held out her hand so I took it to hold
It was ever so tiny and bony and cold
I gave her my trust and I trod where she led
On in the mysterious light that she shed
Half an hour onwards more lights could be seen
Criscrossing the trees' silhouettes were the beams
Of the night traffic passing along the main road
And I barely noticed as faster I strode
Out of the dark wood that her hand had let go
When I turned to embrace her, to gratitude show
I saw nothing to see but a canvas of dark
Where occasional headlights would flash on tree bark

Mortal Memories

Can I to the world bequeath my mortal memories?
Nay, will they even last until I leave it?
If I write this story down in words, can I hope then this
Is a format if they find they can retrieve it

Contact detail

I, Bob Pallister have an Instagram account @randomerbobsxyz that deals with poetry and nothing but poetry. All readers are more than welcome to contact me through this. I also post on the site allpoetry.com, just as Bob Pallister where I can also be contacted.

Acknowledgements

Lots of my fellow poets on Instagram and allpoetry.com have been encouraging about my writing on the subject of my Mum but the one who has been the most supportive is Ruchka a.k.a. @worksadrifing on Instagram. Thank you Ruchka.

Work by Bob Pallister already in print

Les Fleurs du Mal de Charles Baudelaire, The 'Blooms of Badness' Version (Translation) – 2020

100 Metres and Poetry Forms (and Adventures in Writing in Them) 2021

100 Metres and Poetry Forms Further (and Adventures in Writing in Them) 2022

Poems published (6 in total) in two editions of The Cannon's Mouth Poets Quarterly, December 2018 and June 2019

4 poems in the anthology Sun Cycle; Celebrating The World's Season (2019) compiled by Linda Lokhee and Reena Doss.

One poem in collaboration with Big Sal in his 2020 volume The Last Lammergeier

3 poems in the anthology The Pandemic Lockdown Capsized (2020) published by Ink Gladiators Press

26 poems in the Nature Matters, Earth Day Anthology Volume 1 compiled by Kathy Gerstoff

9 poems and 3 invented poetry forms in The 2021 Form runners and Inventors Collection published by Our Earthians Community Group 2021

1 poem in in Ey Up (an Anthology of Northern Poetry) published by Bentkey Publishing in 2022

Printed in Great Britain
by Amazon

13990029R00027